RAGE - Surviving PTSD.

Recognize, Accept, Get Help,Execute

Hendrix Sky

result of the use of the information contained within this document, including, but not limited to, —errors, omissions, or inaccuracies.

Table of Contents

Introduction

You may think that PTSD is a condition that will never affect you unless you serve in the military or witness scenes of warfare. While the condition does affect servicemen, it can also develop after other forms of trauma. The loss of a loved one, the effects of terrorism, natural disasters, or serious injury can all result in PTSD. Trauma is not restricted to a certain type of person. Life is filled with trauma, and until you experience it, you won't know how you will react.

There is no reason to suffer in silence because treatment is available. You can choose natural methods, medications, or therapy. Help could be as simple as improving your diet or lifestyle to work in conjunction with other treatments. Whatever decisions you make, it is important to realize when the disorder is affecting you or someone you know. This book will help you identify the symptoms and triggers that affect sufferers and where and how to seek help.

Part One: Understanding PTSD

Post-traumatic stress disorder is a term we have all heard, but do we really know what it is? Let's analyze the phrase. Post-traumatic - meaning after a deeply distressing or disturbing event or experience. Stress meaning anxiety, worry, or emotional disturbances. Disorder, which means that something's not right, and there is an imbalance in the physical, mental, or emotional parts of your body.

Everybody has experienced trauma of some kind during their lives. It's a fact that life can be brutal, and how we cope with trauma differs greatly from one person to the next. Most of us have developed coping strategies, and with time and self-care, we will recover.

However, sometimes PTSD will follow a disturbing event or experience. Symptoms may appear within a month or even a week following the event, while other subjects have reported a gap of years before experiencing symptoms. Whatever the case, these symptoms can cause significant problems in social and work situations. They can be so severe they interfere with the normal functions we all take for granted.

Generally, the symptoms fall into one of four categories and vary from person to person.

Category 1: Intrusive Memories

These types of symptoms take forms that may include:

- Recurring distressing and unwanted memories of the trauma
- Flashbacks, recalling the event as if it were happening all over again
- Disturbing dreams and night terrors
- Emotional reactions to a reminder of the event, uncontrollable grief or crying
- Physical reactions to reminders of the event like shaking or sweating

Category 2: Avoidance

With this category of symptoms, the sufferer will actively avoid any reminder of the trauma. They will refuse to talk about it and will stay away from places and people that remind them of the event. This can lead to further isolation and become more severe over time.

Category 3: Negative Thoughts and Outlook

Even the most positive people can experience times when they feel a sense of negativity and gloom. That's normal and nothing to worry about, but when these feelings begin to overwhelm someone, it can be hard to regain any form of positivity. If the following symptoms are prevalent, it can be time to seek help for PTSD.

- Negative self-image, believing that everything about yourself is worthless.
- Failure to see any positivity about people around you and the world in general
- Believing the future is hopeless, and there is no point in planning ahead.
- Lack of recall about the traumatic event, distorting facts to alter the result of the trauma
- Difficulty in maintaining formerly strong relationships
- Isolating themselves from family and friends
- Lack of interest in any activities especially ones that were formerly important and part of their daily life
- Lack of positive emotions like happiness or joy
- Feeling emotionally drained and not reacting to outside stimuli.

Category 4: Changes in Emotions

We all react to situations in different ways. For instance, we all have that friend who laughs uncontrollably at the smallest thing and the other friend who takes things way too serious. Some people are prone to emotions more than others, and again that's fine. It would be a boring world if we all reacted the same. However, when emotional reactions change, it can be a sign of PTSD, and treatment may be required.

These are some of the way's emotions can be affected:

- Feeling insecure and being easily startled or frightened.
- Seeing danger in every situation, overanalyzing risks, and the possibility of injury.
- Self-destructive actions, overindulging in alcohol or overeating, driving too fast and taking up dangerous pursuits
- Failure to sleep
- Lack of concentration and tendencies to drift
- Irrational anger and bursts of aggression
- Profuse shame or guilt

One of the most distressing symptoms of PTSD is suicidal thoughts, and any form of this thinking should be addressed immediately. Seeking help from a friend or loved one could be the first step for people who aren't sure where to turn. There is help available from medical sources as well as spiritual sources. Reaching out is the hardest part. If you believe you are about to hurt yourself or you know someone who's in danger, call your emergency number immediately.

After surviving a traumatic event, many people will experience these types of symptoms for a short time.

Most will recover without medical help, but if any of the above symptoms have been occurring for over a month, then it is time to talk to someone who can help.

Failure to address these symptoms may lead to further complications that can disrupt your whole life. Your job, your relationships with others and your personal enjoyment of everyday life will be affected. You are in danger of developing other mental health problems like depression, eating disorders, and substance or alcohol abuse.

The main thing to remember is there should be no stigma attached to PTSD sufferers. It is not a sign of weakness or a lack of character and can affect anybody at any time. Nobody will judge you or believe you are a lesser person if you develop PTSD. The world can be a dangerous place, and we all have different reactions to extreme situations. We are constantly placed under pressure and subjected to extreme high and lows.

Treating early signs of PTSD will help sufferers recover quicker and avoid turning to unhealthy coping methods. Whatever help you need; it is important to open up and tell someone you are having trouble coping. You may find comfort with friends and family who can let you talk about the event or experience and be honest about your reactions. You may need a course of therapy or medication. Understanding you need help, and asking for it is the first step to recovery.

Part Two: Different Types of PTSD

If you have ever experienced a traumatic experience, you will have some idea of the stress that can follow. Life has a way of throwing obstacles in our path and seeing how we cope with them. That's normal, and most of the time, we cope admirably.

However, trauma comes in many forms, and the effect it has on our mental wellbeing can differ. It is estimated that around 8 million adults in the US will experience some form of PTSD during each given year. The number may fluctuate during times of intense stress or when natural disasters occur.

For most people, the disorder is triggered by a serious accident, combat, physical violence, or sexual abuse. Others will suffer PTSD following a sudden loss of a loved one or from witnessing a major event. The people left behind can often suffer from some form of survivor's guilt. They are traumatized by being part of or witnessing an event that has left others dead and has mixed emotions about their own survival.

Of course, not everyone who has experienced trauma will develop PTSD, and it is important to get the right diagnosis before considering treatment. Symptoms will differ for everyone, and some symptoms will not normally be associated with PTSD.

Complex PTSD

This form of PTSD is usually present following a long-term trauma in which the sufferer has been held captive for a prolonged period of time.

This can involve the following situations:

- Being held as a POW (prisoner of war)
- Spending time in refugee camps
- Enforced prostitution or being held as a sex slave
- Forced child labour
- Domestic violence
- Child abuse
- Kidnapping

When experiencing complex PTSD, the sufferer will often encounter feelings of guilt and shame. They will feel responsible for the trauma they have endured and will have a distorted self-perception. They may even experience confusion about the relationship they feel with the perpetrator of the trauma and be occupied with revenge.

They will relive the situation and feel detached from real life. Sufferers will find it hard to trust others and will find it difficult to maintain former relationships.

Comorbid PTSD

This form of the disorder is diagnosed when the patient presents all the criteria for PTSD and exhibits symptoms of other disorders. It is quite common for both men and women with PTSD to present symptoms of depression or some other psychiatric disorder.

Depression has many forms and can range from major depression to bipolar. Situational depression can also be a factor in comorbid PTSD as it is brought on by specific events or situations.

If your case of PTSD has been brought on by the following events, you may be subject to situational depression:

- The death of a loved one
- Developing serious health problems
- Divorce or custody battles
- Domestic abuse
- Physical trauma

Symptoms of depression can vary but will generally present in the following ways:

- Frequent crying
- Feelings of hopelessness and sadness
- Prolonged anxiety

- Change in appetite
- Lack of sleep
- Low energy levels
- Lack of concentration
- Poor body image
- Heaviness in arms and legs for more than an hour at a time
- Sensitivity to criticism

Comorbid PTSD varies so much from person to person and can be difficult to treat as there is no one size fits all solution. It is important to recognize which symptoms are relevant to your situation and how long you have suffered with them.

Dissociative PTSD

This type of PTSD is a recent form that has been associated with people who have suffered early life trauma. Individuals with this form of PTSD exhibit increased heart rate, and decreased activity in the prefrontal region of the brain.

They also experience two other major behavioural problems: depersonalization and derealization.

Depersonalization

The most common symptom of depersonalization is the feeling there is a barrier between the subject and reality. This can lead to the sufferer feeling they are living in a dream world and simply observing the real world. This is your brain's natural defence system kicking in and protecting you from scary things. Prolonged feelings are a symptom of dissociative PTSD.

Depersonalization can also make people feel robotic and lose a sense of their own movements. People who have survived car crashes or other major trauma often report having no recollection of walking away. This is normal, but PTSD sufferers will feel this kind of isolation for longer lengths of time than normal.

Time can also become distorted with depersonalization. Recent events can feel like part of history, and you can feel like you are in a time-lapse. There are gaps and periods where you have no recollection of what happened. This can be disturbing and lead to feelings of despair.

Derealization

This is a mental state which alters your perception of reality. The people you meet or objects around you may seem unreal. They can appear blurry or disproportional, leading you to question their reality. Sounds can also be distorted, and your hearing may seem overwhelmed by the loudness or struggling to pick up any sound at all.

Episodes of derealization can occur for minutes, months, or any other length of time. The sufferer is detaching from reality and retreating to what they perceive to be a safe place. While this may work for short periods, it can be a problem when this behaviour becomes more prevalent.

No lab test can diagnose either of these symptoms, and your doctor will need to test for physical causes. Toxicity in your system may be responsible for behavioural problems, but they can also be brought on by PTSD. An early diagnosis will help you consider what treatment you need and how your condition could be improved.

Part Three: What are the Most Common Triggers of a PTSD Attack?

We have already discussed the symptoms of a PTSD attack and how they differ from one individual to the next. These attacks are often caused by certain triggers. Something happens, or the person finds themselves in a situation that triggers memories of the trauma they have been involved in. This can result in an escalation of symptoms and heightened anxiety.

It is impossible to list all potential PTSD triggers as they can be personal and random to the individual sufferers. Here are some of the most common types of triggers.

Sounds That Can Become Triggers

For a lot of sufferers of PTSD, loud noises and bangs can be one of the most common triggers. Fireworks, firecrackers, vehicles backfiring, and the sound of aircraft can often lead to a PTSD attack. For people who have suffered in an abusive relationship or have had a troubled childhood, it can be the sounds of people yelling or crying.

If you are subject to such triggers, it is important to avoid them in a healthy manner. For instance, if it is New Year or the 1ST of July, try not to go to firework displays or other celebrations that may be loud and raucous. If you are upset by crying and yelling, it may be better for you to avoid crowded restaurants or bars and places where people will show emotion and cause a scene.

Smells That Can Become Triggers

Your memory has an especially strong link to smells, and certain aromas can be key triggers. For veterans that have witnessed horrifying battle scenes and charred flesh, the smell of diesel fuel or meat cooking can be especially distressing.

Other smells can be less obvious. If you have lost a loved one suddenly, then the smell of their favourite perfume or cologne can cause your PTSD to escalate. The smell of food can often be a major trigger when recalling individuals and the times you spent together.

Smells are hard to avoid, especially perfume and other personal aromas, but if you are aware of the scents that are a trigger, you can do something about it. Make sure your friends and family know how much certain smells upset you and ask them not to wear them. If your trigger is burning or cooking meat, then avoid BBQs and other cookout opportunities.

People

For those who are suffering from PTSD, the thoughts of crowds and large groups of people may be enough to make them stress out. This said symptoms could also be triggered by just one person. Maybe you spot someone who has a resemblance to a person responsible for your trauma or who played a part in your rescue. When people die, we often witness such sightings as we subconsciously wish we could see them again.

Similarly, sufferers of PTSD are so desperate not to see anybody who was part of their trauma they can often imagine or hallucinate that they are there. This type of trigger cannot be avoided as it has little basis in truth. Instead, you need to remind yourself that any resemblance is a coincidence and should be treated as such.

It should be noted that sometimes a certain type of person can be the trigger. A policeman or a soldier may bring back haunting images of the trauma and, if possible, should be avoided.

Places

If the location of your trauma was in a hospital or a specific type building, then this can act as a trigger. Of course, you can't avoid hospitals if you are ill, but being aware that it is a trigger that can help you prepare for any future visits. Hospitals and doctors can also trigger an attack with the medicinal smells and sounds that are inevitable.

Circumstances

Being placed in a situation that resulted in trauma can often be a key trigger to a PTSD attack. If you were involved in a serious road accident, you might find that travelling will trigger your PTSD.

The Key Triggers Following a Sexual Attack

This type of PTSD is particularly fuelled by triggers. If a woman has been the subject of rape or a serious sexual assault, their PTSD can be triggered by the presence of a man or even the sound of a male voice. The act of consensual sex with a partner can also trigger serious symptoms of PTSD.

How to Cope with These Triggers

The key to managing PTSD is identifying the triggers and coping with them. This can involve healthy avoidance but should not involve isolation. There is a difference between avoiding fireworks and never leaving the house in case someone lets off a firecracker.

Whenever you experience any symptoms of PTSD, take the time to work out what may have triggered them. Where are you? What can you see or smell? It may be helpful to carry a notebook and pen to record what your triggers are and what helps to ease them.

Try Soothing Your Anxieties

Deep breathing and other meditation exercises can help you become more grounded and bring you back to reality. Your symptoms are taking you to a time that is in the past, and it is important to return to the present. You may have a song that calms you, and having it on hand will help.

You will know what works for you, and you will find a way to use soothing behaviors to feel better. Make sure they are productive and helpful and won't become addictive or harmful. The use of natural soothing behaviours like rocking in a chair or smelling a flower can go a long way to calming your PTSD symptoms.

Part Four: PTSD Treatments

Once the disorder has been diagnosed, your doctor will be able to suggest different forms of treatment. These will be influenced by the history of your trauma and how you are processing it.

The options for treatment include:

1) **Exposure Therapy:** As the name suggests, this therapy includes interaction with key triggers in a controlled environment. The therapist will introduce elements of stress, including people, places, sounds, smells, or images that trigger your negative thoughts and feelings. This form of therapy may seem intense and overwhelming, but it is effective. As the subject learns to control emotional reactions, the effect the triggers have is lessened.

2) **Cognitive Behaviour Therapy:** Normally, this therapy involves one on one talking with a therapist. Essentially, they will help the patient understand how to change their thought patterns and understand how destructive negative thoughts can be. The key part of

changing your behaviour is to change your thought process. There are some helpful online resources available that will enable you to self-help without involving a therapist. Discuss the options available with your medical specialist and decide what works for you.

3) **Transcranial Magnetic Stimulation:** This treatment option involves using images to stimulate the frontal cortex of the patient's brain. Certain symptoms of PTSD indicate an imbalance in the part of the brain that is responsible for certain emotions, including fear and anxiety. Using images to restore the balance will relieve the symptoms with almost no side effects.

   The procedure can also involve using an electromagnetic coil applied to the forehead that administers an electrical pulse to the brain. The strength of the electrical charge is roughly the same as an MRI scan and requires no anesthesia. This will happen if brain imaging is not working, and more intense treatment is required.

4) **Eye Movement Desensitization Reprocessing:** At first glance, this type of therapy seems an unusual way to approach psychological issues. The therapist will help you create a safe place in your mind that you can retreat to in times of stress. They will then use hand motions to distract your eyes while you recall your

trauma. They will guide you to move your thoughts to more pleasant ones with the aid of hand tapping or other forms of distractions. EMDR weakens the effect of negative thoughts and emotions with the distractions they supply when the patient recalls events. Before and after each session, the therapist will ask the patient to rate their levels of distress. As the therapy progresses, it is normal to see these levels reduce significantly. The treatment is effective and can produce results within weeks. Sometimes it will be used in conjunction with other therapies depending on the patients' needs.

Home Remedies for PTSD

While some patients will be encouraged to take medications to treat their symptoms, others will be more comfortable with natural remedies. These types of remedies involve both behavioural and ingested methods of relief.

The following are home remedies you can use to reduce symptoms of PTSD.

Green Tea

While we know that PTSD is a mental disorder, it plays havoc with the body as well as the mind. Green tea will give your immune system a boost and will also reduce anxiety with its soothing properties. You can drink regular tea or add green tea extract to other drinks.

Chamomile

Another soothing form of tea, chamomile, is readily available and pleasant to drink. Chamomile has been used for generations to relax nervousness and reduce negativity.

Valerian

This flowering plant that grows in Europe is a staple part of herbal remedies. It is effective in aiding sleep and treating anxiety, night terrors, stress, and depression. It is sold as an herbal supplement and should be used with the advice of your doctor. It can impair your reactions and should not be taken before driving. Avoid alcohol and other stimulating substances when taking Valerian. Ideally, you should only take Valerian for short periods at a time as it can cause side effects.

Aromatherapy

We all know the power of smells and how they can relax both mind and body. Just as certain smells may induce memories and cause stress, other smells will help you destress. If you are feeling anxious or having a bad day try using lavender or patchouli oil to help you feel less stressed, this type of therapy is based on using distractions. You may find that other forms of distractions work just as well.

Behavioural Remedies

Recovering from PTSD can be difficult and may need a range of treatments. Try these behavioural activities in conjunction with the above natural methods.

Animal Interaction

Many people find that animals help them cope with extreme feelings of anxiety. The use of pets in medical settings actually dates back around 150 years, and the human-animal bond is well documented. Pets can be a beneficial aid for sufferers of PTSD, and interaction with them has proved successful. Check for animal-based therapy courses or simply choose a pet for yourself. Dogs and cats are the most popular, but birds and fish are also great choices as a pet.

Social Engagement

While the natural reaction of sufferers of PTSD is to shut themselves away and avoid interaction, it can be beneficial to engage with others. Actively seeking the company of other people will help you replace your negative feelings of fear with the satisfaction of social engagement. Extended contact with other people will help you realize that life goes on and your problems, while still valid will diminish with time.

Early engagements should be with people who know about your condition and who you trust to react with compassion. As you begin to feel comfortable with them, you can think about progressing to people who are strangers or maybe to bigger groups. As your confidence grows, your anxieties and fears will lessen.

Food and Diet

As the control center of the body, it is important to feed your brain with food that improves mental tasks.

These foods will help your brain stay healthy:

- Fatty fish
- Eggs
- Dark chocolate
- Nuts
- Oranges
- Broccoli

Combined with a healthy diet and regular exercise, your body will be better equipped to deal with your disorder.

Part Five: What Happens When PTSD is Left Untreated?

Many people who suffer from PTSD are inclined to dismiss treatment when they feel they are surviving and managing life to a degree. However, there is both good and bad news for people like these. The good news is that treatment for PTSD is readily available and comes in different forms. The bad news is that PTSD is a progressive disorder, and failure to treat it can lead to co-occurring disorders and other damaging effects.

Untreated PTSD can cause many negative effects on health and well-being, including the following effects:

1) **Eating Disorders:** These types of disorders can occur when the patient has body image issues that result in an obsession with food. Bulimia, anorexia, and binge eating disorder can affect health and can often prove fatal.

2) **Depression:** As PTSD develops, the patient will often suffer from some form of depression.

This can be as mild as chronic depression or as serious as bipolar depression. Untreated depression can affect your life, relationships, and work.

3) **Heart Disease:** Studies have shown that people who suffer from PTSD are more at risk of developing heart problems. It showed that veterans with full-blown PTSD were 5 times more likely to develop heart failure than those who hadn't seen combat. The high levels of stress felt by sufferers are also a major risk factor for heart attacks.

4) **Chronic Pain Disorder:** Sleep disturbance and anxiety can all cause actual physical pain. Headaches, migraines, stomach pain, and muscular strain are all issues that can stem from PTSD. Sufferers are also more likely to neglect their general health, which can also lead to painful conditions like obesity and substance abuse.

5) **Suicidal Tendencies:** PTSD can cause self-harm and suicidal thoughts in its sufferers, and this can cause both mental and physical scars.

How Untreated PTSD Can Affect Your Family and Friends

While a person is suffering from PTSD, they have different levels of control over their life. At first, it may seem that the condition is under control and not affecting other people. The truth is that individuals suffering from PTSD are slowly losing control of thoughts, actions, and behaviours.

Every aspect of life is affected. Relationships are strained as spouses and children are affected. As the disorder becomes more pronounced, work and career prospects will disappear. The patient will experience feelings of worthlessness and self-loathing, which will result in loneliness and isolation.

Spouses often report a feeling of helplessness as they watch their partner descend into a pit of depression and social isolation. Their life lacks purpose, and they are constantly aware that aggression could occur at any point. Spouses and partners of people with PTSD are at risk of breaking down as they feel the person they once loved is slowly disappearing.

Children are also victims of this debilitating disorder. The offspring of sufferers are less likely to do well at school. They often develop at a slower rate than their peers and find it hard to form social ties. They can also display symptoms of aggression or violence that mirror the symptoms of the parent.

PTSD in the Workplace

PTSD is difficult to live within familiar circumstances like the family home, but it can be even worse in the workplace. The key to managing the condition is having patience and understanding. If you are suffering from the condition, it is important to inform the people you work with.

Managers and coworkers should understand that any negative behaviours and impaired work rate could be part of the symptoms and are not entirely in the control of the person involved. However, if the condition is left untreated, it will lead to feelings of resentment if your coworkers feel they are carrying you. Any aggression in the workplace is unacceptable and may lead to problems in the future.

Expect to hear comments about your performance and change in personality; it is part of the disorder. You cannot react with aggression or anger that would be unproductive. Remember your calming behaviours and explain your condition to the other person. If you feel they can help you, then ask for help. People are never as judgmental as you expect, and you will find a measure of understanding.

Sometimes your workplace could be contributing to your condition. If you work in a highly charged atmosphere with career goals and intense workloads, then you may need to rethink your job. The level of success you achieve at work will depend on many factors inside the workplace.

Examples of Work-Related Stress Inducers

1) Unreasonable expectations on employees with the prospect of consequences if they aren't met.
2) Policies that include dismissal for any employees suffering from stress or anxiety. The workplace ethos that both these

conditions show weakness and are not part of an ideal employee.

3) Failure to allow time off for emotional reasons or to deal with periods of stress.

All these policies are part of corporate bullying and will not help people with PTSD to thrive. If you feel your workplace is a toxic environment, you need to report it to a higher source. The days of corporate bullying are hopefully coming to an end.

Research awareness campaigns that deal with PTSD in the workplace and become more informed about the resources available. Take steps to improve your management attitude to PTSD in the workplace and increase their sensitivity.

Workplace culture needs to change, and sufferers of PTSD should expect to be treated with sympathy and respect as they face their condition and seek treatment.

The bottom line is that even though you may feel your level of coping is quite high and you can control your triggers, this may change. Being aware of what the future may hold is a key part of your future decisions. Make other people aware of your condition and ask them to raise any issues they have or any changes they notice. You may miss some details that indicate your condition is getting worse.

Conclusion

Now you know more about the condition, it will be easier to identify if anyone you know suffers from PTSD. Maybe you have encountered trauma or witnessed a life-changing event and are feeling disturbed by your experience? Whatever the case, your new-found knowledge will help you understand how trauma affects people differently. Good luck with your journey, and may you find peace along the way!

Written By: Hendrix Sky

Resources

http://www.lifehacks.com

https://www.health.com

http://www.ourmilitary.com

http://www.calmclinic.com

http://www.curejoy.com

http://www.traumatized.com

http://www.oxfordtreatment.com

http://dailvtrendz.com

www.ingramcontent.com/pod-product-compliance
Lightning Source LLC
Chambersburg PA
CBHW051135250726
48655CB00007B/3083